Is Intuitive Eating More Difficult Than You Think?

The Principles Of Intuitive Eating

By: Wendy Jarich

Table of Contents

Publishers Notes 3

Dedication 4

Chapter 1- What Is Intuitive Eating And How Does It Work? 5

Chapter 2- What Are the 10 Principles of Intuitive Eating? 10

Chapter 3- Does Intuitive Eating Help With Weight Loss? 13

Chapter 4- What Are Common Meal Plans on the Intuitive Eating Diet? 17

Chapter 5- Is Intuitive Eating Healthy? 21

Chapter 6- Does Intuitive Eating Help Obesity Patients? 25

Chapter 7- What Are the Best Superfoods to Eat? 29

About The Author 33

Publishers Notes

Disclaimer

This publication is intended to provide helpful and informative material. It is not intended to diagnose, treat, cure, or prevent any health problem or condition, nor is intended to replace the advice of a physician. No action should be taken solely on the contents of this book. Always consult your physician or qualified health-care professional on any matters regarding your health and before adopting any suggestions in this book or drawing inferences from it.

The author and publisher specifically disclaim all responsibility for any liability, loss or risk, personal or otherwise, which is incurred as a consequence, directly or indirectly, from the use or application of any contents of this book.

Any and all product names referenced within this book are the trademarks of their respective owners. None of these owners have sponsored, authorized, endorsed, or approved this book.

Always read all information provided by the manufacturers' product labels before using their products. The author and publisher are not responsible for claims made by manufacturers.

© 2013

Manufactured in the United States of America

DEDICATION

This book is dedicated to my extremely supportive parents.

Chapter 1 - What Is Intuitive Eating and How Does It Work?

People have been bombing out with their diets for decades now. Today there is a new alternative method for losing weight known as 'Intuitive Eating'. This method relies on the belief that our bodies have good instincts about what we need to eat.

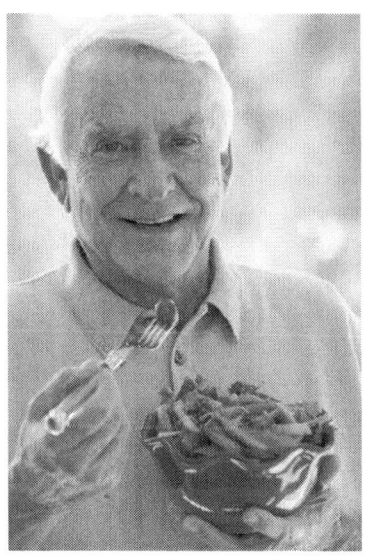

Cravings are not always bad, but can be indicators of what our body is in need of. Nutritionists noticed a barrage of failed dieters coming and going from their offices. They saw the flaws and pitfalls of dieting, and decided to let their clients indulge themselves in some of their cravings. They remained on a strict limited intake, but with this new method they actually lost weight.

This was indeed promising; however, the strict limited intake became a bone of contention. Dieters were unable to stick to the program. That started the nutritionists searching for a totally different approach. After all, the war on obesity had been going on for some time without a lot of progress.

This led to a compromise. It is a new strategy that trades in a program strategy for psychological awareness. It is 'Intuitive Eating'. This method put an emphasis on having the clients increase their sensitivity to their internal signals in regard to hunger and being full. They became more in tune with what they ate and the effects it had on them.

Differentiating

What this method did was to teach the clients how to differentiate between hunger and plain emotional need. They were encouraged to trust in their judgments and natural cravings to work toward a healthier balance.

The permissiveness of this approach really brought the system into question. The experts have mixed opinions as to whether this can really work or not. Some say it clearly cannot be used by everyone. However, there have been thousands of reports stating weight was lost using this exact method. Reviews and studies back up these claims.

The eaters involved in the study showed lower levels of cholesterol, healthier hearts, less diabetes, lower body mass indexes, and higher levels of fitness. This was all done without all the psychological stress that comes with dieting.

With such positive results it is hard to argue there is not something to this. Intuitive Eating really has a chance at a high success rate compared to dieting programs. The experts believe it is because it complements the complex biology that makes up hunger, rather than fighting it. 'Tuning in' seems to work much better than a forced regimen.

Science

There have been some studies done over the past few years that lend credibility to the argument of Intuitive Eating. Before the tests the evidence was mainly testimonial in nature.

It was Tylka who furthered the research concerning Intuitive Eating. She laid down the scientific basis of the research of the eating style and created a scale that could measure and define it.

Her tests laid out 21 traits across 3 broad categories which were-

Unconditional Permission to Eat
Relying on Internal Hunger Cues
Eating From Physical as Opposed to Emotional Cues

and then this scale was applied to over 1,400 people. She determined that Intuitive Eaters possess a higher overall sense of well-being, as well as a lower body weight. They don't seem to be obsessed by the idea of 'being thin'. She also found that of 1,200 college women, a large portion of them shared in a list of empowering traits which were-

Resilience
Optimism
Social Problem Solving Skills
Good Self-esteem

Tylka published a study in 2010 showing that parental pressure on restricted eating during childhood backfired and cause a higher BMI in those people as adults. This pressure backfired because it disconnected people from natural hunger cues. The studies revealed that the adults who participated in the study had a lower tendency for eating when hungry and to stop when they were full.

Hormones

Regardless of what some experts may say about Intuitive Eating, all can agree that traditional diets have failed miserably. They are all largely based on a 'calorie in, calorie out' model. This is a very mechanistic formula that makes the dieter feel as if they are just too lazy or stupid to manage self-control.

Intuitive Eating gives the participants a more positive feeling about themselves and their abilities to handle their weight. That is why this method is getting a lot of review from many experts today.

New research reveals that the stomach along with other critical metabolic parts of our bodies, do not only process food borne calories. They instead are responsible for the sending of dozens of hormonal and chemical messages to our brains. This is where hunger supposedly resides.

Ghrelin is a key hormone in this process. It is the one biomolecule that stimulates our hunger centers in the hypothalamus of our brains. It gets released into our stomachs when it responds to physiological hunger that is triggered whenever cells get short on energy. It also responds to stress and pleasure.

Leptin is another one of our 'safety hormones'. It is produced by the fat cells and lets the brain know it is time to quit eating. Scientists in the past were glad to have discovered Leptin.

The obese, however, have loads of Leptin, and it is not effective in bringing about weight loss. Calorie restriction by dieters only serves to elevate Ghrelin and drives the hunger urges toward overeating and new weight gain. Diets only make things worse.

Consciousness of Eating

Meeting eating desires with a conscious awareness instead of self-will and self-control are that core of Intuitive Eating. Food is everywhere and learning how to become aware of our body's cravings and what they mean, empowers us to exercise some control over it.

Food can be a drug for many people. It stimulates the old serotonin, which is a 'feel-good' neurotransmitter. However, those with enough insight to grasp the concept that the reason they eat is to boost their mood levels, and not because they are hungry, can soon be on their way to solving some serious weight problems. Intuitive Eating could very well be the wave of the future.

Chapter 2- What Are the 10 Principles of Intuitive Eating?

Everyone is looking for the next big craze when it comes to eating right and getting in shape. I'll tell you the ten principles to intuitive eating that will help you live a healthier more energetic life.

The first principle is to respect your body. No one is saying that you need to become a health guru overnight, but there are a few things you can do that they help you improve your quality of life. One of the biggest things you can do to respect your body is to not over indulge in alcohol and cigarettes. In fact, if you can quit smoking this will help and add years to your life. Don't believe the calorie suppressing rumors that come with smoking cigarettes. You can change just a few things that will help reduce your stress without having you rely on this. If you enjoy a cocktail or two from time to time that is fine. Just remember that drinking regularly can add empty calories to your body. Respecting your body can help you enjoy the finer things in life such as family and friends.

The second tip is to embrace your hunger, don't feel like you have to deprive yourself of food just to be healthy and look good. In fact, denying your body of the calories it requires will actually do more damage than good. Ideally you want to eat the right thing and of course know when to stop. When eating out don't feel like you have to clear your plate remember doggie bags are a good thing.

The third principle is to respect your fullness. This relates to the first principle that you don't want to get too full. We all know what when you eat too much to wind up sluggish and exhausted. There is nothing fun about the feeling you get when you've eaten too much, but what do you really gain? The overwhelming need to unbutton your pants; there are a few things you can do to help identify when you're full. Ask yourself how the food tastes if you're losing flavor with every bit it's time to stop.

The fourth tip is to throw away the diet fad. Don't feel like you have to be committed to a book that claims it has the solution you have been searching for instead focus on building a foundation of good solid foods high in protein and vitamins. Discover what you like and don't make yourself feel as if you need to eat something you don't enjoy. Food can be fun so take the challenge to build a strong foundation of good foods and explore you might find something you will learn to love.

The fifth principle is to make peace with food. Food can be fun and instead of fighting it embrace food. If you love to cook these last two principles are perfect for you because you have a chance to love food and rediscover. The best part with making peace is that you can find substitutes that can actually make cooking more fun. Example is to add olive oil instead of butter. Not only will this help you lose weight, but you will be on your way to becoming healthier and notice a burst of flavor.

The sixth principle is related to the last one. You should challenge the rules of good and bad calories. The solution is to have a balance of the two you don't have to be a veggie lover just to be healthy. Yes, that piece of cake isn't totally the enemy, but the trick is to let yourself understand that these desserts shouldn't be an everyday occurrence. Having candy and whatever comfort food you want is o.k., but balance and structure is essential. If you enjoy baking desserts you can find alternative ingredients that can reduce the calories in your favorite snacks so you won't feel so bad. Remember you don't have to torture yourself, but only be nice once in a while.

The seventh principle is dreaded exercise. No one enjoys exercise, but the key is to find something that you enjoy. If you enjoy talking with your friends why not try to walk and talk with them. No matter what type of excise you may enjoy low-impact or high the point is to be active. Get the blood to flow and your heart pumping. So no matter what you enjoy sports, dance, or even playing with your high energy children staying active can really help.

The eighth principle is to learn how to not be an emotional eater. Finding alternative ways to express oneself when you may be upset or angry can definitely help. This one is certainly an easy to say one, but you have to find the willpower and anything else to find a better source to express yourself. Remember that food is only a temporary solution so try to find an interest or hobby to better fill the time. Go see a movie or call up a friend when you're trying to get healthy or loss weight sometime the distraction of a good friend is exactly what you need.

The ninth principle is to discover the satisfaction factor. Finding what you really want to eat and not just what is available can help you feel more fulfilled and less willing to eat more than you have too. When you find what you really want your body can tell you when to stop eating and you don't end up over eating.

Finally, the tenth principle is honor your health this is related to the first principle where you should respect your body. Knowing your health and what your history can help you with losing weight, feeling healthy, and becoming the best you. When you honor your health you will see that your family will want to follow as well.

Now that you know the ten principles you can apply them and find a healthy new you.

Chapter 3- Does Intuitive Eating Help With Weight Loss?

Learning how to tune into your body's physical and emotional cues is essential for maintaining your health. When you learn how to recognize your body's signs that it is in need of care, then you will be better able to realize when you are sick, overtired or even hungry. Intuitive eating is based upon the principle that a person should become an expert regarding how their body works. It also includes the belief that everyone is born with the innate ability to recognize the signals of hunger and that no food should be classified as good or bad.

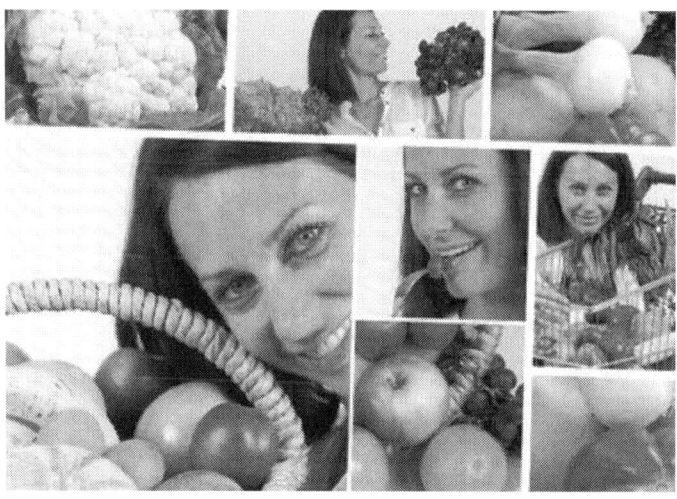

Throughout their lives, many people have learned unhealthy eating habits that have led to increased weight gain, fatigue and other health problems that could be avoided if they did not overeat. Those who have been shamed regarding their eating habits may also have begun to associate negative emotions with their eating such as guilt or depression. The intuitive model of eating eliminates these negative connotations so that you can begin to experience the benefits of healthy eating habits. If you are ready to embrace the idea that you can have control over your body, then here are a few benefits that you should know regarding how intuitive eating can help with weight loss.

Eliminates the Negativity of Dieting

When most people think of dieting, they often associate it with deprivation. However, starving your body of the nutrients it requires will only lead to binges and further health problems. Diets may lead to rapid weight loss in the short-term, but most of the weight is gained back as soon as someone falls off the diet wagon. To compound matters, diets are usually too rigid to provide the nutrition a person needs to stay healthy. Many of them are too strict to comply with on a daily basis. As you begin to practice intuitive eating, you will begin to recognize the lies that exist in every crash diet claim you have ever heard.

Learn to Respond to Hunger Signals

Starvation diets never work, because they lead to overeating to fulfill the insatiable hunger that results from going too long without eating. When you starve your body, it also holds onto the fat out of a biological need to create reserves in case the body is truly starving. By learning to recognize the first signal your body sends that it is hungry, you will be able to eat smaller meals without the fear of binging. Hunger pangs, growls and a desire to eat can all be cues that it is time to fuel your body with a healthy meal.

Develop a Positive Attitude Regarding Food

Learning to stop the voices of the food police is a primary component of intuitive eating. For many people, food has negative connotations that influence the types and amounts of food they select. Forbidden foods have a tendency to create a stronger urge to binge on them due to the guilt that is created every time they are consumed. Instead of categorizing foods as bad for you, you will learn to recognize how certain foods affect your body. Surprisingly, many people discover that their favorite foods only cause them to feel worse or can lead to a crash in their energy. This discovery intuitively guides people to healthier options when they are planning their meals.

Conquer Emotional Eating

As you become more self-aware, you will also begin to be able to identify the emotional triggers that play a role in your dietary habits. It is common for people to eat more in response to negative emotions such as anger, boredom or sadness. Instead of trying to fill these holes in your emotional make up with food, you will learn how to acknowledge them as normal. Then, you will begin to implement positive coping methods that can take the place of food for making you feel better.

Find Pleasure in Food

After years of dealing with the constant cycles of dieting and overeating, many people have stopped finding pleasure in food. However, food is a wonderful thing that causes many enjoyable sensations to be felt while eating. As you begin to create a calm environment for your meals and eat according to your body's signals, you will start to notice the wonderful sensations that accompany your food. Being mindful of the aromas, tastes and textures of your food will enable you to feel pleasure even if you are eating less.

Know When You Are Full

Overeating occurs when a person eats beyond their physical need for food. During the process of transitioning to intuitive eating, you will take brief breaks to assess your fullness level. As you eat, ask yourself if you are feeling satiated, overly full or still need to eat some more. As long as you listen to your body's signs, you will recognize the fulfillment of your hunger so that you eat less every time.

Respect Your Physical Self

When a person does not feel good about their body, it can be too easy to give up and just overeat. Through intuitive eating, you will learn that your body is a work in progress that is unique. This means that no matter how much you weigh or what your size may be, you are exactly who you should be at the time. As you begin to respect your body, you will also want to care for it through giving it the nutrition it requires to stay healthy and active. This healthy attitude regarding your body will also serve as inspiration for exercise.

Finding ways to overcome the negative associations you have with eating will provide many benefits across all areas of your life. Intuitive eating is designed to teach you how to listen to your body so that you can identify the signals it is sending. By learning how to eat only when you are hungry while avoiding the emotional triggers that spur overeating, you will begin to enjoy food once again while making progress toward a healthy body and weight loss.

Chapter 4- What Are Common Meal Plans on the Intuitive Eating Diet?

Those who embrace intuitive eating often like to say that they are not using a diet plan at all; they are not eating just specific foods or sticking to a set of rules that dictates what they are allowed to consume. Instead, they are just using common sense and paying attention to the things that their bodies want and need. The result is a healthy lifestyle that can help them lose weight, even though their meal plans could look vastly different from someone else who is using the same technique to control the foods that they eat.

The basic principle behind the plan involves paying attention to your body. Are you hungry? If so, go ahead and eat. That is just your body telling you that you need food. Are you starting feel full? If you are, stop eating. You do not need to keep going just to clean your plate or to continue eating in a social setting. If your body is telling you that you have had enough, you should stopping adding more calories to your diet. When you do this, you can really slash your total calorie count and get your weight back under control.

Another big aspect of the diet or eating plan is that you should not eat snacks unless you are hungry for them. Many people eat for emotional or mental reasons. For example, you might eat ice cream if you are feeling sad, or you might eat a bag of chips while watching television because you are bored. If you added up those snacks, which your body never asked for, you would have thousands of extra calories. Getting rid of them is a big step toward making yourself feel healthy and looking your best once again.

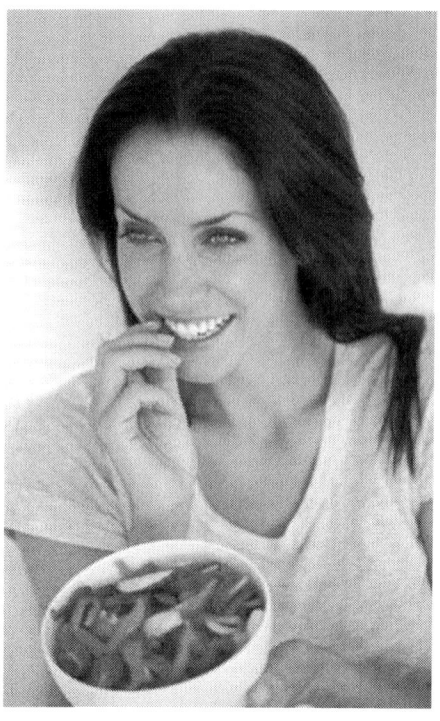

The result of this process is that, even though you are allowing yourself to eat anything that you want, you are eating far less. You are using common sense. How often have you stuffed yourself for no reason? It is one thing to overeat on a holiday, when it is at least expected, but you have probably done it at random times as well. Everyone does. Even though you are just eating by yourself and you are as full as you need to be, you might keep going just for something to do. This is ignoring your body's signals, and it leads to weight gain more than eating unhealthy foods.

That being said, meal plans do not exist in the traditional sense. For a standard diet, your meal plan could consist of actual types of food. You might eat nothing but an English muffin or a piece of fruit for breakfast. For lunch, you might have vegetables or tuna fish. For dinner, you could have a bowl of steamed vegetables. With some diets, you might even replace one of those meals with a shake or a drink. This is a very structured way to eat, and people often make the mistake of thinking that it is the only way to lose weight.

In reality, though, this can make you gain weight. You are going to break your diet, and when you do, it is going to be bad. You are going to stuff yourself with food. This is the body's natural reaction. It thinks that you are running out of food, due to the reduced meals, and it is trying to get you extra calories in case you are living in a drought or a famine. It is hard to fight these urges, which are buried deep inside of everyone from years of human society and evolution.

An intuitive meal plan should not be so structured. Instead, it should be more of a general mindset that you use whenever you come to the table. You should start with small portions and make sure that you drink at least one glass of water while you eat. Always remember to eat your food slowly, which gives your body time to figure out when it is really full. Packing in food as quickly as you can means that you could go far over your intended calorie count long before you realize that you have already had plenty of food to eat.

This mindset will drive the way that you eat, regardless of what you are having. If you make a pizza for your family, just eat one piece and then see how you feel. Are you satisfied? You may be surprised to find, in a world in which people often eat three to four pieces of pizza in one sitting, that you really do not need more than one. You did not force yourself to eat nothing but lettuce and fruit, so you got to enjoy your meal, but you could still come in at 500 to 1,000 calories less than someone who ate too much.

Your meal plans should include healthy foods when possible. It is always better to eat fruits and vegetables than foods that are high in fat content. This diet is not a way for you to give up on salads and start eating pizza and ice cream all of the time. Instead, it is just a way for you to regulate and control yourself. If your plan includes healthy foods eaten in modest amounts, giving your body the calories that it needs without going overboard, you can start to see a positive impact on your overall weight.

One trick that people sometimes use is to have healthier meal plans during the week and then really let themselves have extras on the weekends. This is dangerous because you could overeat by a lot on the weekends, but it can also be helpful. It is very hard not to eat an extra piece of cake when you do not know the next time that you are going to get one. It is far easier to pass on one on a Tuesday when you know that you can have it without any guilt on Saturday.

Chapter 5 - Is Intuitive Eating Healthy?

Listen to your body and how it feels when you eat certain foods. Does a certain type of food make you feel sick? Are you more energized when you have a big breakfast and then eat smaller portions of meals throughout the day? By listening to your body and eating what you want you are practicing a form of intuitive eating. This method of eating involves giving in to your desires and eating what you want. You should pay attention to how your body and mind reacts to eating certain types of food.

This eating style is not designed to allow you to indulge into eating any type of food that pleases your taste buds. You are supposed to listen to your body and mind after eating food to determine which makes you feel the healthiest and function the best throughout the day. This can mean eating certain types of foods, a particular amount of times each day, or consuming certain portion sizes. It may sound like a carefree diet but there are actually a number of principles that you need to follow in order to properly practice intuitive eating.

The first step involved with intuitive eating is to get rid of thoughts of how you view traditional diets. Most people follow a 2,000 a day calorie diet. The truth is some people need more than 2,000 calories a day, while others may need less. This is where the second principle of the practice of eating comes into play. The most important part of intuitive eating is to listen to your hunger. Eat until you feel satisfied.

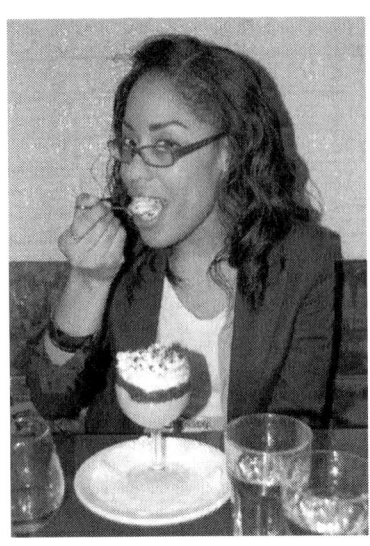

This does not mean that you should finish your plate; eat only enough to help your stomach feel comfortable. The next step might sound a little much but it is necessary to feel comfortable with what you are eating. You need to feel comfortable eating every food that you put into your stomach. Eat what you want as long as you do not overdue it. It makes no sense to finish an entire bag of chips just because you were bored. Following intuitive eating does allow you to add a portion of chips to your meal or to eat a portion as a snack. Pay attention to your body before you eat any food. Are you truly hungry? This is where people mistake hunger for cravings. You may eat foods that you want but only if you are actually hungry.

The fourth principle involved with intuitive eating is to avoid the traditional sense of portion sizes. Bigger people naturally need more food while smaller people can only handle a certain amount of food. Reaching fullness after every meal to promote a healthier body is the fifth principle to follow. Failing to reach fullness won't allow you to nourish your body properly with food and energy to function. Becoming satisfied after a meal is the sixth principle and is important to understand as well. Eat a mixture of food that includes something to fill your belly; foods with the right amount of vitamins. You want to satisfy your hunger and at the same time eat proper nutrition.

One of the most important principles to follow is the seventh. Never eat as a result of stress anxiety, anger, or other emotions. Your goal should be to eat to nourish your body and at the same time satisfy your hunger. It is fine to eat sweets but that does not mean you should eat unhealthy. The next time you go to the kitchen to get ice cream before bed, think twice. Are you really eating the ice cream because you are hungry or are anxious about the day ahead? Are you sad about something that happened that day? Listen to your emotions and only eat when you are hungry and not as a reaction to your feelings. Practice this principle and you should not have a problem with your eating habits.

The last steps to follow are to respect your body, exercise, and honor your health. The eighth principle outlines that you should feel comfortable inside your body. Some people are just going to naturally be skinnier or bigger than others. As you respect your body make sure that you also exercise regularly. Stop worrying about following a workout routine designed by another person. Listen to your body during and after a workout. Exercise until you feel like comfortable with the workout you completed. The last principle is to practice healthy eating habits. You know what is good and what is bad for you. Fill your meals with healthier foods regularly. Research and learn about the types of foods that are good for your body. Visit your doctor to receive a physical and evaluation. Listen to suggestions on what you should add and take out of your diet on a daily basis.

Intuitive eating is only healthy when you do not have an eating disorder of any kind. People that eat way too much or too little every day can wind up to become very unhealthy. Before you decide to commit to intuitive eating get checked out by a doctor. Overweight people should still try to manage the food they eat so that they do not put their health at risk.

Someone that has been anorexic in the past or that does not eat the right amount of food every day should try to eat a healthy amount of food. Intuitive eating can be healthy as long as you are not tricking your mind. There biggest problem people face with this diet is they do not know the difference between hunger and cravings. A craving is when you have the desire to eat food even though you are not hungry. When you eat in this fashion it can prove to be unhealthy. Intuitive eating promotes the idea of only eating when your body is hungry. So in truth this way of eating is actually a very healthy practice.

Chapter 6 - Does Intuitive Eating Help Obesity Patients?

To understand the way that intuitive eating can help those who suffer from obesity, you first have to look at exactly how it works. Generally speaking, this is a diet plan that tells you to stop thinking about dieting. Rather than concentrating on eating less or trying to cut calories, you should simply stop worrying about it and just eat whatever your body desires. Make sure that you only eat when you are hungry, but do not force yourself to eat a salad when you get hungry; if you want ice cream, just eat ice cream and enjoy it.

The theory says that this will work for two reasons when trying to cut back obesity. First of all, it keeps you from eating when you are not hungry. Many people eat snacks as part of an event, rather than a meal. For example, you might order a pizza when you are going to watch the Super Bowl just because you know that the two often go together. You might buy a bag of candy when you are going to the movies. You do not need these foods, so these are all wasted calories that make you gain weight. By doing away with them, you can drop the extra pounds.

The other side of the theory is that you really desire some of those unhealthy foods just because you are always trying to diet. The act of denying them makes them more attractive than they would be otherwise. For instance, you might really love chocolate ice cream. When you crave it and you eat a piece of toast instead, you just crave it more. It becomes something more attractive than it would be otherwise precisely because you are telling yourself not to eat it. When you finally break down and indulge yourself, then, you eat two or three times as much as you would have otherwise.

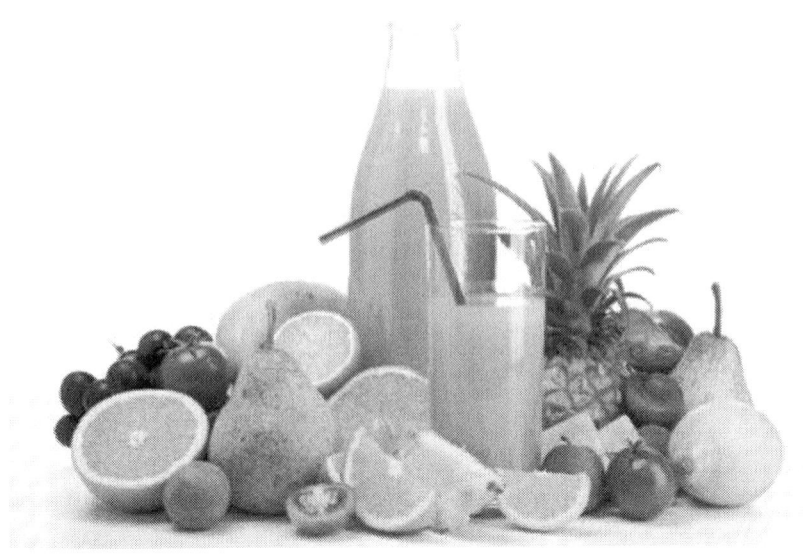

A good example of how the change could work is if you start eating just one spoonful of ice cream every single day. This makes it a normal occurrence, something that is part of your routine. In between spoonfuls, you do not really crave the ice cream. You know you are always going to get some more. It is not forbidden. If you put it off for a week, you might pat yourself on the back and then eat a huge bowl as a reward, giving yourself far more calories than you would have gotten in the seven spoonfuls.

There is evidence that this intuitive eating plan can certainly help those who are obese. It will likely be ineffective right at first, though. People who are just starting out are still in the "dieting" mindset. They finally feel free, and they eat a lot of food as a result. Do not expect this to have good results overnight. It takes some time for you to work through this initial stage and actually start to see the good results that you have been after.

However, this is how it is supposed to work. Go ahead and eat a bowl of ice cream every day for a week. Have pizza for dinner every night. Pretty soon, you are going to get sick of it. Since it will now be allowed in any amount that you want, it loses some of its charm. You will start choosing other, healthier options of your own free will. Those things that you thought of as vices will become things that you do not really care about anymore. This is when you can start to transform the way that you eat and begin to lose weight.

As is shown, this is more of a mental diet than a physical one. You have to realize how your brain is tricking you into eating too much. By changing the way that you think about food, you can change the way that you use it. While a traditional diet takes a lot of will-power and can be very hard, which is why people often struggle to diet for years, never losing more than a few pounds, an intuitive eating plan is not hard at all, so you can still sustain it even after you start to lose weight.

The hardest part is probably going to be eating only when you are hungry. Modern culture attaches food to many different things. When you think about the holidays, what do you think of first? On the Fourth of July, you eat pie and hot dogs. On Thanksgiving, you eat more pie and turkey. On Christmas, you eat cookies and drink egg nog. Every holiday seems to have a food attached to it, no matter how minor it is. This even holds true for other events, such as birthday parties and, as mentioned above, sporting events or trips to the movies.

These are the times when you need to control your eating. Tell yourself to get back to the way that the human body was designed to work. Eating was originally for nothing more than sustaining the body. Since people often lived through famines, they got used to eating as much as they could when they had food, storing up for the months or years when there was not enough to go around. Now, you have plenty of food all of the time, so you have to fight your body's natural training. Put those snacks aside and just eat when you really need food.

Finally, there can be some other side effects of this plan that you will enjoy. For example, putting off your diet will reduce the stress that you feel. Did you know that stress can cause you to gain weight? An intuitive eating plan can help you break this cycle. You will also be happier with the way that you are living, not feeling like you are trapped in a world where all of the good foods that your friends are eating are denied to you. You can just relax and enjoy your life while losing weight.

Chapter 7 - What Are the Best Superfoods to Eat?

Most people eat because they enjoy the sensation of tasting the food versus eating for the proper nutrition. The sad truth is that most of the foods that we enjoy eating and taste good are the ones that have no health benefits to them. If a nice, big cheeseburger helped you lose weight and boosted your immune system, our world would be the healthiest world ever. Sadly, it does not work that way, and we have to think about what we are putting in our mouths if we want to be healthy.

If you want to have optimal health, your diet is going to play a major role. Your personal health is a good reflection of what goes into your body and how you live your overall life. Even though those pre-packaged processed foods are nice and convenient, cooking your food from scratch with unprocessed fresh ingredients is the best way to have optimal health.

You have probably heard the word "superfood" buzzing around in recent years, and several of the processed food products claim to have superfood ingredients. Never let those claims fool you. When foods are processed, it denatures the nutrients. What you end up eating is something with less quality compared to the real food product. It is always better to stick with whole organic foods.

Listed below are some of the best superfoods you can eat. These whole foods offer many nutrients you should implement into your balanced diet. Incorporate as many of these in your diet as you can on a weekly or daily basis for the best start. Remember, all the superfoods on this list are either organic or wild.

Organic Pastured Eggs – Pastured eggs, also known as free-range eggs, are a great source of nutrients that a lot of people are deficient in such as fat and high-quality protein. One single egg contains nine amino acids, high quality protein, lutein and zeaxanthin, choline and naturally occurring B12. Ideally, it is better to eat the eggs as close to raw as you can (poached or soft-boiled). As long as you buy good organic eggs that are fresh, you can eat them raw and not worry about getting salmonella. Pastured chickens are a lot healthier than farm chickens and are low risk for infections.

Kale – Kale is a cruciferous vegetable that is very inexpensive and helps relieve chest congestion. It is very beneficial for your immune system, liver and stomach. It provides a great source of nutrients and vitamins including vitamins A, B and C, calcium, lutein, zeaxanthin, iron and chlorophyll.

Yogurt or Raw Grass-Fed Kefir – To help increase your energy and boost your immunity system, add some kefir or yogurt made from raw milk that is grass-fed to your diet. Kefir is a fermented food full of probiotics, a very healthful bacterium. It cannot be stressed enough how important it is to have a healthy gut flora. Probiotics do more than just help your body digest food; they influence your genes to help them behave in a disease-fighting manner. The friendly bacterium helps your immune system prevent the trigger of allergies. Probiotics will help your weight normalize. Pasteurized food and drinks will not give you the same benefit. The abundance of phosphorus in kefir helps to utilize fats, carbohydrates and proteins that promote cell growth and energy.

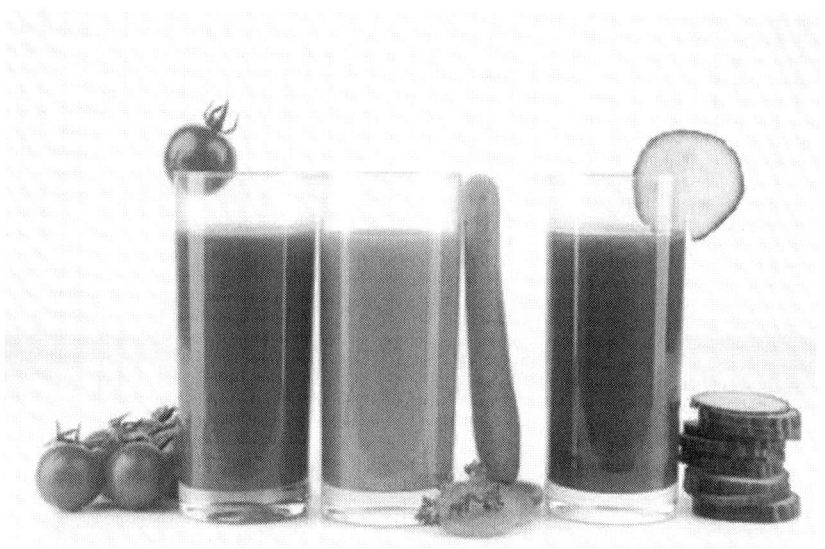

Raw Organic Almonds – Almonds are a great source of whole foods as long as they are raw. Raw nuts are full of polyunsaturated and monounsaturated fats. These fats are a good way to promote a healthy cholesterol count. They have no trans fats as long as they are not pasteurized. Raw almonds are a great source of phytochemicals which promote a healthy heart. They are a good source of iron, fiber, protein, phosphorus, magnesium, calcium, vitamin E and potassium.

Wild Alaskan Salmon – Wild Alaskan salmon is full of nutritional benefits. It has high levels of DHA, EPA and omega-3 which most people need in their diets. Alaskan salmon is a great source of high-quality protein, antioxidants, astaxanthin and essential omega-3 fats.

Avocados – Most Americans are deficient in the healthful raw fat found in avocados. Avocados offer the body over 20 healthy nutrients including B-vitamins, vitamin E, fiber, folic acid and twice the amount of potassium you find in a banana. Additionally, an avocado enables the body to absorb fat-soluble nutrients.

Organic Coconut Oil – Half of the content of fat in coconut oil is a fat that is rarely found in nature, lauric acid. Lauric acid is known as a "miracle" ingredient because of its natural health promoting properties. Inside the body, the lauric acid is converted into monolaurin. Monolaurin has anti-bacterial and anti-viral properties. In addition, the saturated fats found in this coconut oil promote better heart health, weight loss, support the immune system, support a good metabolism and give you an instant source of energy.

Coconut oil increases activity in the thyroid as well. Perhaps one of the most interesting benefits of coconut oil is the potential it has for warding off dementia. For cooking, coconut oil is a great choice. It is the only oil that will resist heat-induced damage because it is stable. One or two tablespoons of coconut oil added to your diet a few times a week will do wonders.

Green Vegetable Juice – Making vegetable juice with your veggies is the best way to have a sufficient amount of vegetables in your diet. Drinking raw vegetable juice is like having an intravenous infusion of enzymes, minerals and vitamins going right into your body without having to break down. There are plenty of benefits of organic vegetable juice. It can help with weight loss efforts, boost your immune system, increase your energy and support brain health.

Superfoods have been around for years. Recently they have really gone main stream. Several food products are based around them, and diet experts sing the praises of incorporating superfoods into your diet. They help you resist disease, make you healthier and give you more energy. Why not incorporate these superfoods into your diet today?

About The Author

Wendy Jarich began eating things such as Tofu, which has been used in Asian cooking for thousands of years and is now becoming more popular in vegetarian cooking and mixed in with dishes for meat lovers. The soft curd can be substituted for cheese and meat and is like a sponge as it soaks in flavors of other ingredients. Tofu is full of nutrients, easy to digest and not expensive so it is cheap so a great way to bulk up meals and save some money too.

Wendy Jarich also uses olive oil as one that has numerous qualities that chefs both amateur and professional favor. Studies show it is a great appetite suppressant and can give a feeling of being full which means you are less likely to over indulge. It's ideal as a salad dressing, cooking oil or on bread instead of using butter or margarine. Add some balsamic vinegar for a tasty treat.

Printed in Great Britain
by Amazon